MEDITERRANEAN DIET FOR BEGINNERS

Your Essential Guide to Living the Mediterranean Lifestyle

Adele Baker

Disclaimer

The recipes and information in this book are provided for educational purposes only. Please always consult a licensed professional before making changes to your lifestyle or diet. The author and publisher shall have neither liability nor responsibility to anyone with respect to any loss or damage caused or alleged to be caused directly or indirectly by the information contained in this book. All trademarks and brands within this book are for clarifying purposes only and are owned by the owners themselves, not affiliated with this document.

Images from shutterstock.com

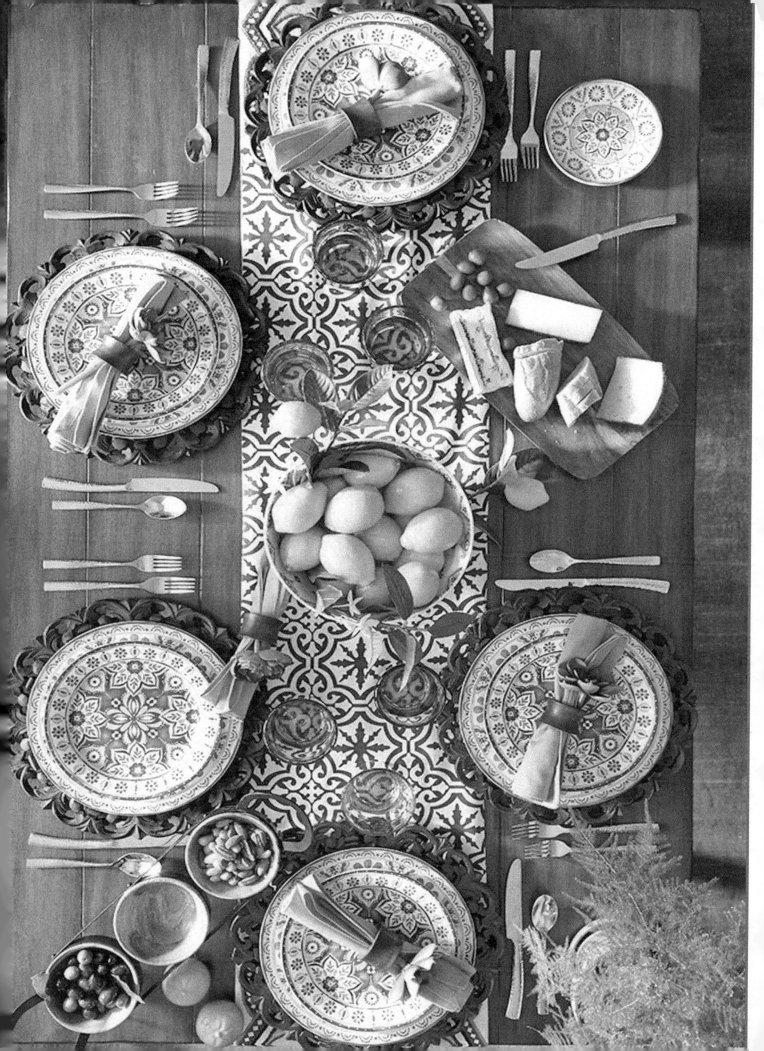

Your Gift

By joining my newsletter, you will be notified when I release a new book and be able to buy it for a reduced price.

Now you will get for free **TOP recipes for any occasion from the best-selling author Adele Baker.**

All files will be delivered to your inbox (in PDF format) and can be read on your laptop, phone, or tablet.

Just click the link below to signup and receive your free book:

http://www.adelebaker.com/promo/recipesfortwo_IS

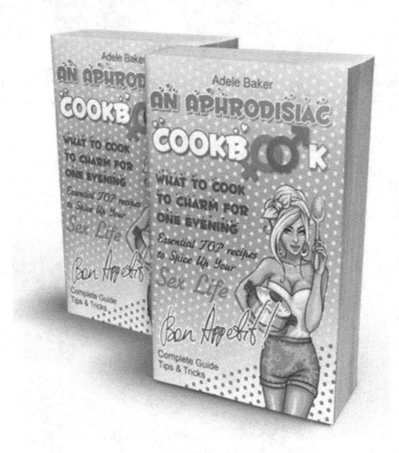

I know you will love this gift!

Thanks, and enjoy!

CONTENTS

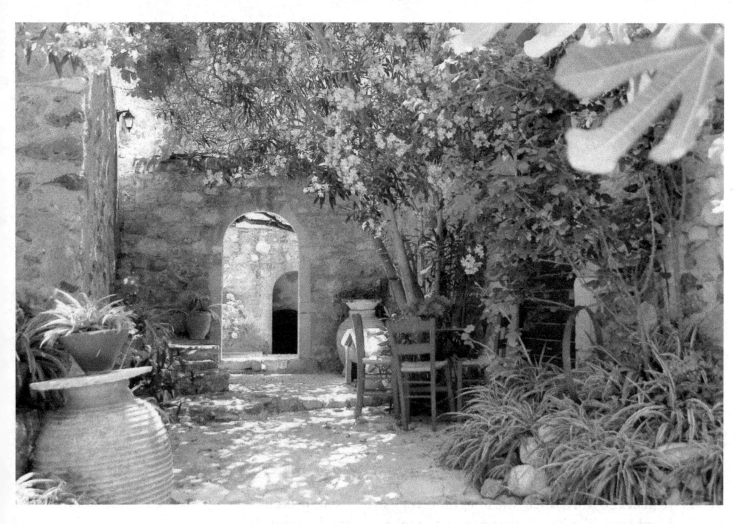

INTRODUCTION

Have you ever dreamt about a diet without a strictly written menu for every day, starving and forcing yourself to follow all the rules? Can you imagine a well-balanced diet that offers tasty and diverse food while at the same time boosts your health and keeps your fit? Believe it or not, the Mediterranean diet meets all these parameters and is considered to be one of the healthiest dietary patterns in the world. In addition, it is more a formula of nutritious food and a kind of lifestyle than a strict list of what you can and cannot eat.

The Mediterranean diet is associated with consuming fruits, vegetables and grains, limiting fats, replacing salt with herbs and spices, eating fish and poultry instead of red meat. It may even include a glass of red wine per day, and regular physical activities to see the remarkable health benefits. The Mediterranean diet reflects various eating habits of the countries near the Mediterranean Sea, mainly Southern Italy, Greece, France, and Spain. Being not just a diet but a set of skills, knowledge, and traditions, it has been found to prevent heart attacks, reduce the risk of depression and dementia, and aid in weight loss. So, if you are struggling with excess weight, you should definitely try the Mediterranean style of eating.

It is essential for you to know all aspects of the diet you are going to take up. This book will provide you with all necessary information including the basic points of the Mediterranean diet, history of its development, key ingredients, good advice for beginners and plenty of recipes. It is highly likely that after reading this book, you will see a plate of healthy, colorful, and delicious food according to the best principles of the Mediterranean diet on your dinner table.

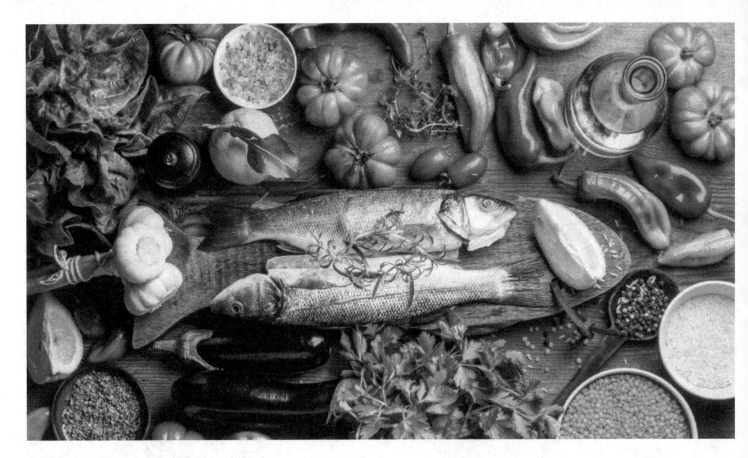

What is the Mediterranean Diet?

When we hear the word "diet," we imagine a very strict list of products we are allowed to eat. On the other hand, the phrase "the Mediterranean diet" makes us think about the sea, long beaches, fresh air, and exotic fruit. This image is really inspiring and gives a good start to understanding the Mediterranean diet.

To start with, the Mediterranean diet is not technically a usual diet – it's a long tradition of nutrition and lifestyle habits of some cultures near the Mediterranean Sea. There is even an opinion that the Mediterranean diet is not a diet at all, it's a lifelong habit, something you should accept as a creed. Italy, Greece, Spain, and France – all these countries have their own exquisite cuisine, but they share some common eating principles, like fresh seasonal food, and these foods appear to be very useful and healthy. According to several health studies, the average life expectancy of people living in this region is longer than in other areas in the world. Also, these inhabitants suffer less chronic heart diseases, diabetes, cognitive decline, mood disorders, and other health-related problems.

Everyone realizes the great importance of well-balanced nutrition for our health, but because of the crazy rhythm of modern life, very few people actually manage to follow a healthy diet, and tend to find simple and easy variants when it comes to meals.

The Mediterranean diet doesn't involve anything extraordinary or difficult, it doesn't even require any supplements. With this dies, there is an emphasis on fresh fruits and vegetables, whole grains, nuts, seafood, and replacing unhealthy fats with olive oil. In contrast to some other diet plans, the Mediterranean way of eating doesn't limit any products or food groups; it mainly encourages eating different foods moderately. It's important to eat small amounts of food but support its high quality. It will be very nourishing and at the same time will keep you from overeating. This is why the Mediterranean diet is also very effective for those struggling with obesity. You can achieve your weight loss goal while enjoying a delicious meal.

Here are the general principles of the Mediterranean diet:

- Increase intake of organic and seasonal fruits and vegetables.
- Substitute butter and margarine with extra-virgin olive oil.
- Replace white flour with whole grain flour.
- Eat fish and shellfish three or four times a week.
- Eat low-fat milk, cheese, and yogurt.
- Use nut butter instead of dairy butter.
- Only eat red meat and pork a few times per month.
- Use nuts as shacks.
- Drink one or two small glasses of red wine per day.
- Eat three or four eggs per week.
- Do physical exercise!

The Mediterranean diet has been proved to be one of the healthiest diets known to man. This way of eating is worth following, even if switching from fast food to fish and low-fat milk seems difficult to you. Maybe some diet plans do not meet your expectations despite all the promises and big words. But rest assured, the Mediterranean diet will make a difference if you make the effort. It will keep you healthy and happy!

History of the Mediterranean Diet

The principles of the Mediterranean diet come from the dietary traditions of as the people in Italy, France, Greece, Portugal, Spain, and Cyprus. This diet reflects various cultural peculiarities while creating its own rich system of lifestyle principles. The Mediterranean diet is quite possibly most established eating routine on the planet, with three thousand years of history.

The main components of this diet were formed through the centuries. A great number of Mediterranean people worked as farmers, cultivating grapes and olives. Some of them were fishermen. In the Mediterranean, people didn't consume beef or dairy products because of unsuitable climate conditions for these kinds of animals.

It is not a new diet, and maybe that is exactly what makes it so popular and widespread. Even after centuries, this way of eating has remained completely unchanged, keeping all crucial principles and components.

Among the scientists who studied the Mediterranean diet was Dr. Ancel Keys. In 1958, he began examining heart-healthy diets and lifestyles. Over fifteen years, in seven nations, Dr. Keys researched disease and mortality rates.

The result of his study showed that the death rate in Mediterranean countries was lower compared to the US. He concluded that the main reason for the difference was lifestyle and eating traditions.

An expanding number of studies have shown the favorable effects of the eating regimen followed in the Mediterranean region. They also confirm that this diet lowers the level of obesity, heart problems, and Type 2 diabetes.

The Road to Health Improvement

The Mediterranean diet has anti-inflammatory components, plant-based foods, and low-fat products. But physical exercise and not smoking are also essential to achieve prosperity.

Though heavily based on fruits and vegetables, this diet still allows for a chance to eat, drink, and be happy. Here are some of the privileges of following this eating pattern:

Decreases heart-related problems

The Mediterranean diet has proved to help relieve the symptoms of some chronic illnesses and heart-related problems. It decreases the rate of cardiovascular mortality because of its favorable effect on "bad" cholesterol – the low-density lipoprotein which carries all fat molecules around the body in the extracellular water. An impressive impact of the Mediterranean diet on heart health is also due to olive oil. The Warwick Medical School has revealed that people consuming more extra-virgin olive oil have lower blood pressure than those eating sunflower oil.

Red wine in moderate amounts, another component to this diet, has also been shown to reduce heart diseases.

Protects against Type 2 diabetes

Compared to vegetarian diets, vegan diets, and high-protein diets, the Mediterranean diet is more beneficial for people with diabetes or high blood sugar. Plant-based food and olive oil decrease blood sugar and cholesterol. The Mediterranean diet contains little sugar because it comes only from fruit, wine, and the occasional dessert.

Promotes healthy weight loss

The Mediterranean diet is a suitable method of maintaining your weight without starving and watching calories. Studies have discovered that consuming olive oil rather than products packed with unhealthy fat makes your body spend more calories. According to German scientists, even the smell of olive oil enables you to feel fuller during the day and intuitively eat fewer calories. So, the Mediterranean diet can act as a natural appetite suppressant. Managing weight gain and loss is easier while on the Mediterranean diet because portions are smaller than in the typical American's diet.

Lower the risk of developing Alzheimer's disease

The Mediterranean diet has a positive effect on blood pressure and blood vessels. Providing us with antioxidants, it will prevent chronic inflammation in the brain and entire body. Thus, it reduces the chances of suffering from dementia or Alzheimer's disease. This kind of nutritional plan also gives aging adults an opportunity to keep their life activity and works against cognitive decline.

Helps to avoid Parkinson's disease

Fruit, vegetables, olive oil, and seafood dishes rich in antioxidants protect your cells and help to avoid damage that causes diseases like Parkinson's.

The Mediterranean Diet Pyramid

General guidelines of the Mediterranean diet are gathered in the Mediterranean Diet Pyramid. It is accepted to be the "gold standard" dietary plan that boosts your health.

The pyramid was created in 1993 and gave the Mediterranean diet tremendous popularity. It was developed by the Harvard School of Public Health and Oldways Preservation and Exchange Trust, an organization specializing in healthy nutrition promotion.

The pyramid reflects social and cultural traditions of the Mediterranean lifestyle. It is more than just arranging food in order of their relative importance — it explores the principles of choosing, cooking, and serving food. The portion sizes and food quality also need special attention.

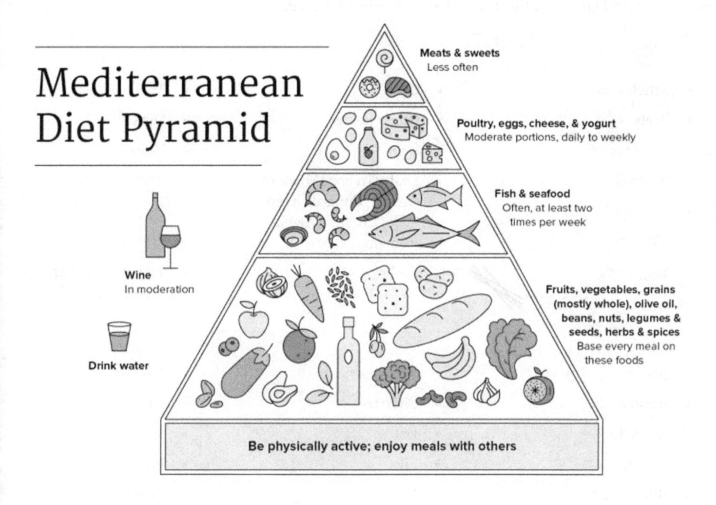

The base of the pyramid shows the great importance of strong social connection, exercise, and sharing meals with your family and friends. You should put a priority on active exercises such as running and aerobics, and even small things like housework or walking up the stairs can contribute to your health.

One of the biggest sections of the Mediterranean Diet Pyramid is devoted to plant-based food. Fruits and vegetables, beans, whole grains, olive oil, nuts, herbs, and spices are the most important components, so you should consume them every day. Eat fresh and seasonal food, avoiding processed food as much as possible.

Moving upward, there is fish and seafood. In the Mediterranean region, they usually have fish two times a week. Eggs, cheese, yogurt, and poultry are also included in the Mediterranean eating plan; they are encouraged in moderation. Red meat and sweets are not eaten very often or only in small portions.

Wine can be had, but in moderation and usually with meals, about one or two glasses per day. Wine is known to improve heart health, protect and strengthen the immune system, and reduce the risks of dementia. The other essential component of the Mediterranean Diet Pyramid is water. It's necessary for proper digestion, and good for your body overall.

Together, these components can have a strong impact on your mental and physical health. They promote the development of a profound appreciation for the delight of eating healthy and tasty meals.

Main Ingredients

Here is a typical grocery list to kickstart your Mediterranean diet:

Vegetables

- Artichokes
- Beets
- Bell Peppers
- Broccoli
- Cabbage
- Carrots
- Eggplant

- Garlic
- Green Beans
- Kale
- Leafy Greens (Mustard Greens, Collard Greens, Swiss Chard, Arugula, Romaine)
- Leeks

- Mushrooms
- Olives
- Onions
- Peas
- Squash
- Spinach
- Tomatoes (Fresh, Canned, Sauce)

Fruits

- Apples
- Apricots
- Avocados
- Bananas
- Blueberries
- Cranberries

- Strawberries
- Cherries
- Dates
- Figs
- Grapes
- Lemons

- Melons
- Oranges
- Peaches
- Plums
- Pomegranates

Beans

- Black Beans
- Chickpeas (Garbanzo)

- Lentils
- Pinto Beans

- White Beans (Cannellini)

Grains

- Barley
- Bulgur
- Couscous
- Oatmeal
- Pasta
- Polenta
- Quinoa
- Rice

Herbs and Spices

- Anise
- Basil
- Bay Leaves
- Cilantro
- Clove
- Coriander
- Cumin
- Fennel
- Lavender
- Marjoram
- Mint
- Oregano
- Parsley
- Pepper
- Pul Biber
- Rosemary
- Sage
- Savory
- Sumac
- Tarragon
- Thyme
- Zatar

Nuts and Seeds

- Almonds
- Cashews
- Flax
- Peanuts
- Pine Nuts
- Pumpkin Seeds (Pepitas)
- Sesame Seeds
- Sunflower Seeds
- Walnuts

Seafood

- Clams
- Cod
- Crab
- Salmon
- Scallops
- Shrimp
- Tilapia
- Tuna

Healthy Oils/Fats

- Avocado Oil
- Canola Oil
- Extra-Virgin Olive Oil
- Grape Seed Oil

Dairy/Eggs

- Cheese
- Low-Fat Milk
- Plain or Greek Yogurt
- Eggs

Let's have a close look at some key ingredients and their health benefits.

Chickpeas

Chickpeas provide our body with fiber. Some researchers have found that fiber protects from colon cancer, helps to fight diabetes, and prevents heart-related problems. Chickpeas are rich in magnesium, iron, zinc, calcium, and vitamin K, and support bone structure and strength. In turn, vitamin C and vitamin B-6 reduce heart disease risk.

Olive Oil

This important ingredient of the Mediterranean diet brings several significant health benefits. Oleic acid, the main monounsaturated fatty acid in olive oil is considered to lower inflammation and suppress genes related to breast cancer. Famous for its strong anti-inflammatory properties, olive oil is shown to decrease the risk of heart disease, diabetes, Alzheimer's, and obesity. Olive oil can also destroy or decrease the rate of harmful bacteria. One of these is Helicobacter pylori, a bacteria in stomach that is thought to cause stomach ulcers and even cancer.

Almonds

Studies suggest that consuming almonds considerably boosts the level of vitamin E in the plasma and red blood cells, and also decreases cholesterol levels. Almonds have been found to have a positive effect on levels of blood lipids and to improve heart health. Nut consumption reduces the risk of breast cancer by 2–3 times.

Garlic

Garlic is famous for its capacity to boost the immune system because it contains vitamin C. This vegetable also helps to avoid cardiovascular diseases by reducing blood pressure.

Eggplant

Eggplant helps to maintain bone structure and protect from osteoporosis. This vegetable contains no fat or cholesterol and contains fiber, which helps us feel full. Among other useful abilities of eggplant is boosting brain activity and general mental health. This is due to phytonutrients that increase blood flow to the brain, improving the powers of memory and analytic thoughts.

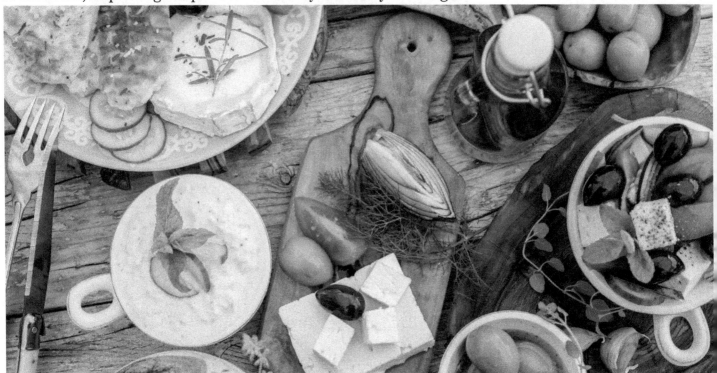

The Pros and Cons of the Mediterranean Diet

Every diet has some drawbacks and certain components that could cause harm to your health. So, before adopting a new dietary pattern, you should check with your doctor.

Advantages of the Mediterranean Diet:

1. The diet promotes longevity and boosts health.
2. It's rich in delicious recipes and gives you more meal options than other plant-based diets.
3. Includes various healthy fats and oils.
4. Basic components are whole, fresh, seasonal foods.
5. You don't need to restrict or starve yourself.

Disadvantages of the Mediterranean Diet:

1. Is not recommended for hyper-sensitive system.
2. You should check all criteria of the diet before you actually start it. Make a list of qualities of the eating plan that are advantage or disadvantage for your health. Every diet for that matter has some qualities that align with certain body type and system. This should influence your choice of diet a lot. For example, hyper-sensitive system or suffering from an ailment can make the Mediterranean diet an inappropriate choice.There is no set amount of food or types of food that need to be consumed per day.

How to Make this Diet Work for You
The Top Ten Hints for Your Success

When starting something new, we all expect immediate results and that we will achieve our goals quickly and without too much effort. Such expectations usually cause frustration and disappointment, and we make a quick conclusion that the plan isn't suitable for us. That's the main reason why people give up on many diets. Firstly, you must believe in your success and make an effort to improve your health. Secondly, implement changes to your lifestyle gradually and they will become long-term habits.

To get as many health benefits as possible from the Mediterranean diet, mind these tips and incorporate them into your everyday routine.

1. Active lifestyle

The Mediterranean lifestyle encourages eating healthy foods, but exercise is also a big part of their way of life. At home, you can play with the kids, clean the house or yard, walk with your dog in the park, skate, or ride a bike more and drive less, and take the stairs instead of using the elevator. When you go shopping, park as far from the building, if it's possible. It will make your trip a few minutes longer, but later you will notice positive changes in your body.

2. Enjoy your meals with family

Start planning family dinners more often, at least twice a week. Besides having fun moments, you will also bring some benefits to your health. Don't just pick up some fast food to bring home, get your children involved and spend a great time together cooking a healthy, homemade meal. This will give you a chance to become more creative. Surprise your family with something new and tasty.

3. Substitute butter with healthy oils

Try to use extra virgin olive oil or canola oil instead of butter or margarine. If your recipe includes an unhealthy fat, replace it with the same quantity of olive oil. This will be useful for your heart, and at the same time the dish will become even more delicious. Consuming olive oil and limiting butter, mayo and other saturated fats is a main principle of the Mediterranean diet.

4. Use more spices and herbs, avoiding salt

Herbs and spices are rich in antioxidants, which raise the nutrient value of meals and reduce sodium levels. On the other hand, some researches have revealed that salt increases blood pressure. You can also use sea salt instead.

5. Use plant-focused recipes

Meat is usually the main focus in dishes in the USA, but the Mediterranean diet encourages using more vegetables. Fruits and vegetables are the core components of this eating pattern, so it is better to put them in the middle of your plate rather than on the side.

For dessert, choose fruit, but add honey or brown sugar to get some special flavors. Instead of crackers or chips, eat fresh fruit as a snack.

6. Consume more fish instead of red meat

For the Americans, it's sometimes difficult to eat fish two times a week and avoid red meat. Nevertheless, this principle of the Mediterranean diet has tremendous importance because it has anti-inflammatory properties. Fatty fish like herring, salmon, sardines, or tuna may serve as an appropriate replacement of meat.

7. Eat more legumes

Legumes are a crucial component of the Mediterranean diet. They substitute for meat perfectly. Beans are high in minerals and antioxidants and a huge source of protein and fiber, so they help you to lose weight.

8. Substitute refined flour with whole grains

Eat whole grain products instead of foods like white bread and white rice. Try quinoa, barley, or millet. Such foods are perfect for a healthy breakfast and have significant nutritional value.

9. Drink alcohol moderately

It's typical for Mediterranean people to drink red wine with meals. Try not to drink outside of mealtime, and not to excess.

10. Eat seasonal food

Shop at the local farmers market for fresh seasonal products. Make eating a special ritual, and don't let yourself eat in front of the TV or while surfing the web.

Mistakes and Misconceptions of Beginners

Although the principles of the Mediterranean diet are familiar to a great number of people, some misconceptions still exist. Here are the most widespread myths about the Mediterranean diet.

Myth 1: Being on this diet is expensive.

Fact: If your dietary plan includes mainly beans, grains, and some seasonal vegetables, it is actually cheaper for you to eat this way than consuming processed or fast food.

Myth 2: The diet is unhealthy because of fats and oils.

Fact: A core component of the Mediterranean diet is oils, but that doesn't make it high-fat. This eating plan encourages consuming heart-healthy monounsaturated fats like avocado oil, extra-virgin olive oil, and canola oil.

Myth 3: The Mediterranean traditions include large portions of pasta and gyros.

Fact: Yes, pasta is a typical Mediterranean food, but portion sizes differ from those in the USA and is mainly serves as a side dish. Vegetables and fish are usually the main components.

Myth 4: Drinking wine as much as you want is the Mediterranean way.

Fact: The Mediterranean people don't actually drink a lot of wine. It's good to consume one or wo small glasses, but more can bring some unpleasant healthy consequences. The main thing here is moderation.

Myth 5: Eating a lot of cheese is fine.

Fact: Eating a lot of cheese can increase the daily dose of calories and saturated fats you take in, so your weight goals may not come true.

Myth 6: You don't have to limit yourself in sweets and desserts.

Fact: People in the Mediterranean region usually have dessert for special occasions and in small portions.

Myth 7: You don't have to change your lifestyle and habits.

Fact: Full adoption of the Mediterranean diet requires some additional time for shopping, cooking, and serving. It's important to slow down your life rhythm, rest, and enjoy the company around you more.

BREAKFAST

Oatmeal with Yogurt & Egg

Prep time: 3 min

Cooking time: 2 min

Servings: 1

Nutrients per serving:

Carbohydrates –46 g

Fat – 9 g

Protein – 17 g

Calories – 320

Ingredients:

- ⅓ cup oats
- ⅓ cup low-fat milk
- 1 egg
- ¼ teaspoon cinnamon, ground
- ¼ cup yogurt
- ¼ cup apple, slashed
- Salt, sugar to taste

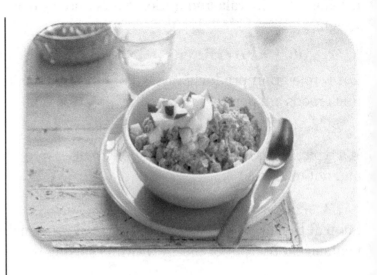

Instructions:

1. Blend the milk and egg. Mix in all ingredients except yogurt and apple.
2. Microwave until the liquid is evaporated, (for about 2 minutes).
3. Spread yogurt and apples on top of oatmeal.

Baked Eggs with Spinach

Prep time: 10 min

Cooking time: 20 min

Servings: 4

Nutrients per serving:

Carbohydrates –4 g

Fat – 7 g

Fiber – 2 g

Protein – 10 g

Calories – 120

Ingredients:

- 4 eggs
- 1 package frozen spinach, defrosted, chopped
- ¼ cup Cheddar cheese, shredded
- ¼ cup chunky salsa

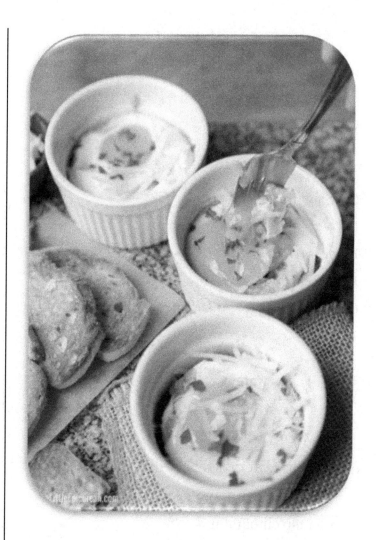

Instructions:

1. Preheat oven to 325°F.
2. Put equal amount of spinach into 4 custard cup. Make a well in the middle by pressing down with your fingers.
3. Add an egg into each indentation. Spoon salsa and shredded cheese on the top.
4. Cook for 20 min.

Quinoa & Dried Fruit

Prep time: 5 min

Cooking time: 15 min

Servings: 4

Nutrients per serving:

Carbohydrates –44 g

Fat – 7 g

Fiber – 6 g

Protein – 13 g

Calories – 285

Ingredients:

- 3 cups water
- 1 cup quinoa, rinsed
- ¼ cup walnuts
- 8 dried apricots, halved
- 4 dried figs, large
- 1 tsp cinnamon

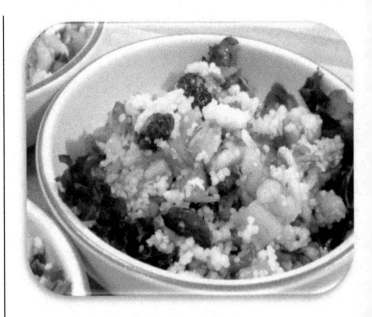

Instructions:

1. Combine quinoa and water in a pot and let simmer for 15 minutes, until the water evaporates.
2. Chop dried fruit.
3. When quinoa is cooked, stir in all other ingredients.
4. Serve cold. Add milk, if desired.

Eggs & Hash & Cheese

Prep time: 3 min

Cooking time: 3 min

Servings: 1

Nutrients per serving:

Carbohydrates –7 g

Fat –14 g

Protein – 15 g

Calories – 210

Ingredients:

- 1 egg
- ½ cup hash browns, shredded, frozen
- 2 Tbsp cheese, cheddar or feta
- Salt & pepper, to taste

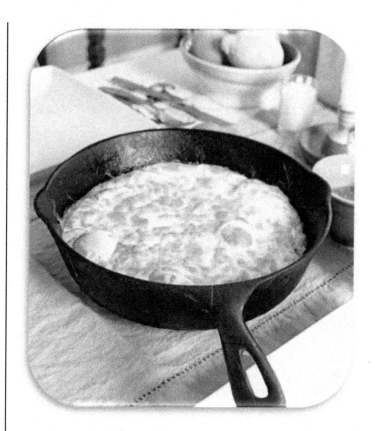

Instructions:

1. Grease a microwaveable bowl with olive oil spray and fill with hash browns. Microwave for 1 minute, and add salt and pepper to taste.
2. Stir in an egg and beat well. Microwave for 45 seconds.
3. Sprinkle cheese over the top.

Veggie Breakfast Bowl

Prep time: 2 min

Cooking time: 3 min

Servings: 1

Nutrients per serving:

Carbohydrates – 2 g

Fat – 6 g

Fiber – 1 g

Protein – 10 g

Calories – 100

Ingredients:

- 1 egg
- 1 Tbsp water
- 2 Tbsp mozzarella cheese, shredded
- 2 Tbsp mushrooms, diced
- ¼ cup baby spinach, thinly sliced
- 2 Tbsp cherry tomatoes

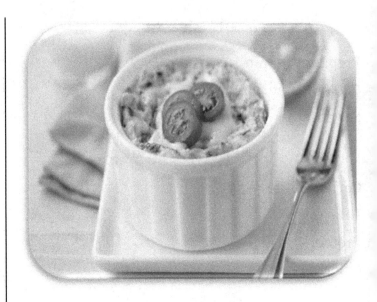

Instructions:

1. Combine all ingredients except for the cheese in a greased microwaveable bowl.
2. Microwave for 1 minute or until the egg is cooked.
3. Sprinkle shredded cheese over the top.

Apple Peanut Butter Oatmeal

Prep time: 10 min

Cooking time: 8 hours

Servings: 4

Nutrients per serving:

Carbohydrates – 50 g

Fat – 11 g

Fiber – 7 g

Protein – 10 g

Calories – 320

Ingredients:

- 1 cup steel cut oats
- ¼ cup brown sugar
- ½ tsp cinnamon
- ¼ cup peanut butter
- 1 tsp vanilla extract
- 2 apples, diced
- Salt, to taste

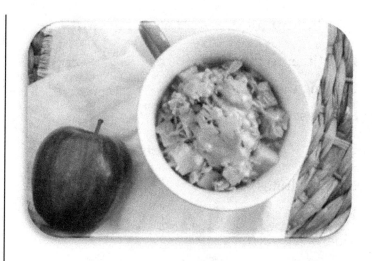

Instructions:

1. Grease a slow cooker with cooking spray.
2. Add all ingredients to the crockpot except apples, mix well.
3. Add apples to the top of the mixture and cook on low for 8 hours.

Edamame & Sweet Pea Hummus

Prep time: 10 min

Cooking time: 15 min

Servings: 2

Nutrients per serving:

Carbohydrates – 35 g

Fat – 30 g

Fiber – 5 g

Protein – 20 g

Calories – 460

Ingredients:

- ½ cup edamame, cooked
- ½ cup peas, cooked
- 2 Tbsp tahini
- 1 clove garlic, minced
- 2 Tbsp mint, chopped
- 3 Tbsp extra-virgin olive oil, divided
- 2 wheat tortillas
- 2 eggs

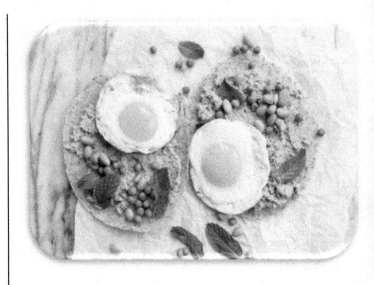

Instructions:

1. Blend first 5 ingredients and 1 Tbsp of olive oil in a food processor. Spread evenly over the wheat tortillas.
2. Coat pan with remaining olive oil and cook the eggs. When ready, put one egg on each tortilla.

Muffin Pan Frittatas

Prep time: 10 min

Cooking time: 15 min

Servings: 6

Nutrients per serving:

Carbohydrates – 3 g

Fat – 10 g

Protein – 12 g

Calories – 165

Ingredients:

- 6 eggs
- ½ cup milk
- 1 cup cheddar cheese, crumbled
- ¾ cup zucchini, chopped
- ¼ cup red bell pepper, chopped
- 2 Tbsp red onion, sliced
- Salt & pepper, to taste

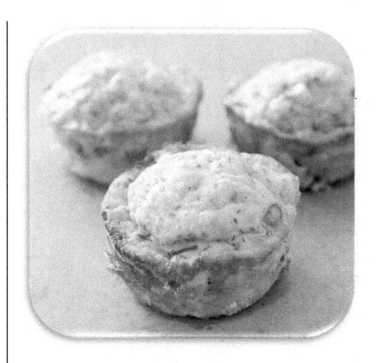

Instructions:

1. Preheat oven to 350°F.
2. Whisk together the eggs, milk, salt, and pepper. Then mix in other ingredients.
3. Spray a muffin tin with cooking spray and distribute the prepared mixture evenly between the cups. Bake for 15 min.

SOUPS, SALADS & SANDWICHES

Avocado Pasta Salad

Prep time: 20 min

Cooking time: 0 min

Servings: 6

Nutrients per serving:

Carbohydrates – 50 g

Fat – 10 g

Protein – 8 g

Calories – 300

Ingredients:

- 3 Tbsp marmalade
- ⅓ cup juice, orange or tangerine
- 1½ Tbsp extra-virgin olive oil
- 2 small oranges, sliced
- 1 Tbsp white wine vinegar
- 2 tsp Dijon mustard
- 1 avocado, diced
- 1 sweet red bell pepper, chopped
- 4 cups pasta, cooked
- 3 onions, sliced

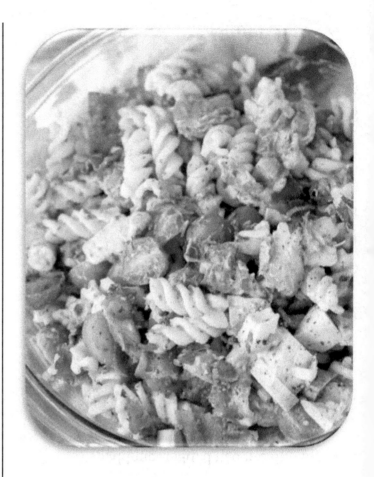

Instructions:

1. Mix together the juice, marmalade, mustard, oil, and vinegar.
2. Stir in pre-cooked pasta. Let chill.
3. Mix in remaining ingredients.

Cretan Salad

Prep time: 20 min

Cooking time: 15 min

Servings: 4

Nutrients per serving:

Carbohydrates – 55 g

Fat – 13 g

Fiber – 7 g

Protein – 17 g

Calories – 380

Ingredients:

- 4 potatoes, cut into cubes
- 3 boiled eggs, cut into quarters
- 2 zucchinis, sliced
- 2 cucumbers, sliced
- 2 tomatoes, sliced
- 1 onion, sliced
- ½ cup Greek olives
- ½ cup lemon juice
- 4 ounces of Greek feta, cubed

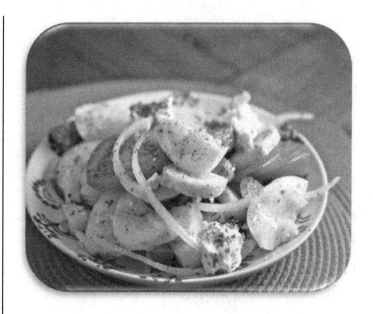

Instructions:

1. Boil and chill potatoes and zucchini.
2. Mix all ingredients and season with salt and pepper.

Black Bean & Mango Salad

Prep time: 20 min

Cooking time: 15 min

Servings: 4

Nutrients per serving:

Carbohydrates – 25 g

Fat – 7 g

Protein – 8 g

Calories – 180

Ingredients:

- ½ cup mango, diced
- 1 cup canned black beans, rinsed
- ½ cup red pepper, diced
- ½ cup lentils, cooked
- 1 cup jalapeño pepper, minced
- ¼ cup onion, minced
- 2 tbsp. cilantro, minced
- 4 tbsp. orange juice
- ½ tsp. sea salt
- 2 tbsp. extra-virgin olive oil

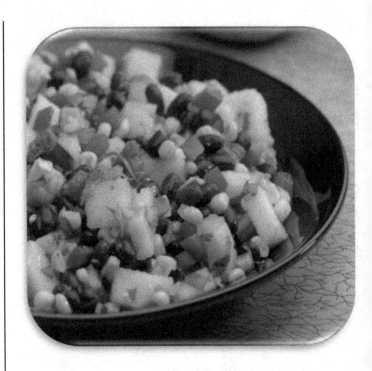

Instructions:

1. Prepare lentils and let cool.
2. Mix together all ingredients and serve.

Summer Strawberry Salad

Prep time: 10 min

Cooking time: 0 min

Servings: 6

Nutrients per serving:

Carbohydrates – 25 g

Fat – 18 g

Fiber – 5 g

Protein – 4 g

Calories – 260

Ingredients:

- 1 cup Kalamata olives, halved
- 5 ounces lettuce, rinsed
- 1 cup strawberries, quartered
- ½ cup dried pitted dates, chopped
- ½ cup blue cheese, crumbled
- ½ cup candied walnuts

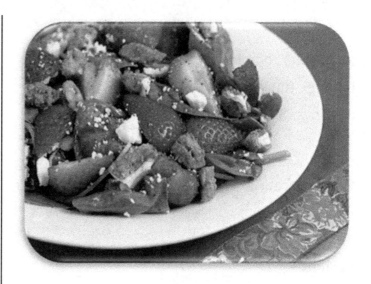

Instructions:

1. Arrange lettuce on a plate, and top with remaining ingredients.

Walnut & Cucumber Gazpacho

Prep time: 10 min + 1 hour

Cooking time: 0 min

Servings: 8

Nutrients per serving:

Carbohydrates – 15 g

Fat – 24 g

Fiber – 4 g

Protein – 5 g

Calories – 275

Ingredients:

- 4 English cucumbers, chopped
- 1 bunch scallion, chopped
- ½ bunch mint
- ½ bunch parsley
- ½ red onion, peeled
- ⅓ cup champagne vinegar
- ½ cup olive oil
- 6 ounces low-fat yogurt
- 1 cup walnuts

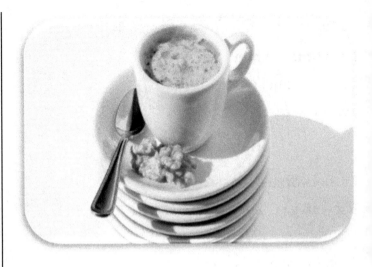

Instructions:

1. Season cucumbers with a pinch of salt and let rest for 1 hour.
2. Combine everything in a blender and blend until smooth.
3. Season with lemon oil.

Cretan Lentil Soup

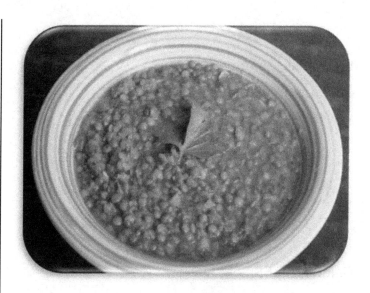

Prep time: 20 min

Cooking time: 45 min

Servings: 6

Nutrients per serving:

Carbohydrates – 25 g

Fat – 36 g

Fiber – 5 g

Protein – 10 g

Calories – 450

Ingredients:

- 1 pound lentils, without stones
- 6 cups water
- 1 cup extra-virgin olive oil
- 1 onion, grated
- 3 carrots, grated
- 2 cloves garlic
- 1 slice orange, peeled
- 2 Tbsp tomato paste
- 1 bay leaf
- Salt & pepper, to taste

Instructions:

1. Combine lentils and water to a large pot. Boil for about 15 min.
2. Stir in the rest of the ingredients and cook on low for 30 min.

Smoked Salmon Sandwiches

Prep time: 10 min

Cooking time: 0 min

Servings: 4-8

Nutrients per serving:

Carbohydrates – 7 g

Fat – 5 g

Protein – 6 g

Calories – 168

Ingredients:

- 4 grain rolls
- ¼ cup feta
- 4 ounces smoked salmon
- 1 cucumber, sliced
- Several leaves baby spinach
- Several sprigs fresh dill

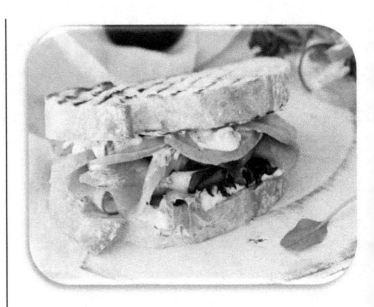

Instructions:

1. Halve the rolls.
2. Arrange them on the counter and distribute cheese on each bread half.
3. Put a piece of salmon, cucumber, some lettuce and dill on the top of each helping.

Red Pepper & Avocado Tartine

Prep time: 10 min

Cooking time: 0 min

Servings: 2

Nutrients per serving:

Carbohydrates – 55 g

Fat – 18 g

Fiber – 7 g

Protein – 6 g

Sugar – 11 g

Calories – 430

Ingredients:

- 4 slices bread, toasted
- ½ cup Greek-style yogurt
- 1 roasted red pepper, chopped
- ¼ tsp black pepper, cracked
- 1 avocado, sliced
- ½ tsp za'atar seasoning

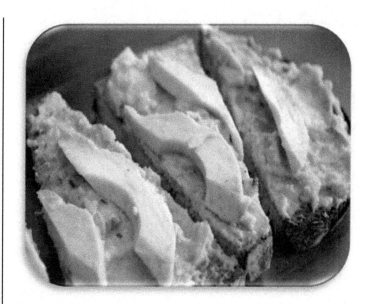

Instructions:

1. Combine pepper and yogurt in a bowl, seasoning with the black pepper.
2. Spread the mixture equally on each slice of toast. Top with a slice of avocado.
3. Use za'atar seasoning, if desired.

SNACKS

Peanut Butter Popcorn

Prep time: 15 min

Cooking time: 5 min

Servings: 4

Nutrients per serving:

Carbohydrates – 56 g

Fat – 20 g

Fiber – 6 g

Protein – 9 g

Calories – 430

Ingredients:

- 2 Tbsp peanut oil
- ½ cup popcorn kernels
- ½ tsp sea salt
- ⅓ cup peanuts, chopped
- ⅓ cup peanut butter
- ¼ cup agave syrup
- ¼ cup wildflower honey

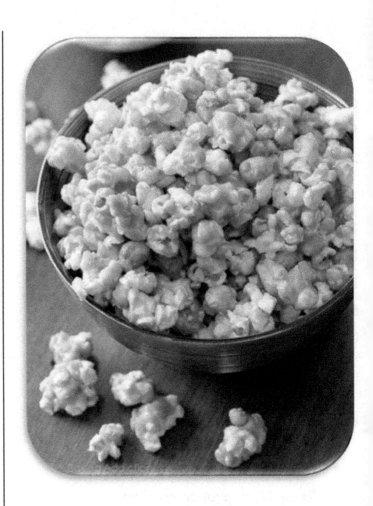

Instructions:

1. Combine popcorn kernels and peanut oil in pot.
2. Over medium heat, shake the pot gently until all corn is popped.
3. In a sauce pan, combine the honey and agave syrup. Cook over low heat for 5 min, then add the peanut butter and stir.
4. Coat the popcorn with prepared sauce.

Greek Yogurt

Prep time: 10 min

Cooking time: 0 min

Servings: 2

Nutrients per serving:

Carbohydrates – 90 g

Fiber – 10 g

Protein – 16 g

Calories – 380

Ingredients:

- 1 cup nonfat Greek yogurt
- 2 oranges
- 4 to 6 Medjool Dates, chopped
- 2 Tbsp honey
- 2 Tbsp pistachios, chopped

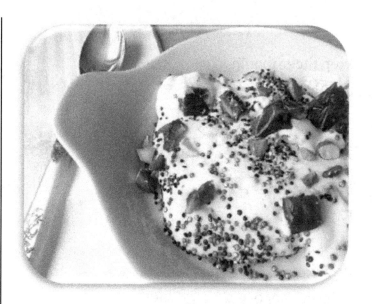

Instructions:

1. Arrange orange slices in bowls, making semicircles.
2. Top oranges with yogurt.
3. Garnish with honey, pistachios, and dates.
4. Let cool in the fridge for a few hours before serving.

Avocado & Blueberry Bang

Prep time: 10 min

Cooking time: 0 min

Servings: 2

Nutrients per serving:

Carbohydrates – 40 g

Fat – 13 g

Fiber – 15 g

Protein – 4 g

Calories – 250

Ingredients:

- 1 frozen banana, peeled, chunked
- 2 avocados, quartered
- 2 cups berries (use your favorite combinations of blackberries, strawberries or raspberries)
- Agave or maple syrup, to taste

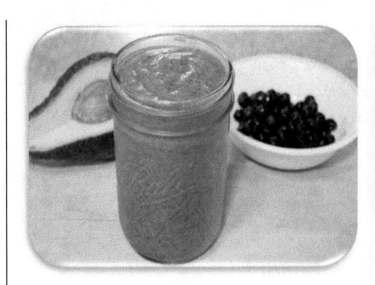

Instructions:

1. Blend all ingredients except agave or maple syrup. Add ice water, if needed.
2. Garnish with syrup and serve in smoothie glasses.

Parmesan Herbed Walnuts

Prep time: 15 min

Cooking time: 30 min

Servings: 8

Nutrients per serving:

Carbohydrates – 4 g

Fat – 21 g

Fiber – 2 g

Protein – 8 g

Calories – 220

Ingredients:

- ½ cup Parmigiano-Reggiano cheese, grated
- ½ tsp Italian herb seasoning
- 1 tsp parsley flakes
- ½ tsp garlic salt
- 2 cups walnuts
- 1 egg white
- Cayenne pepper, to taste

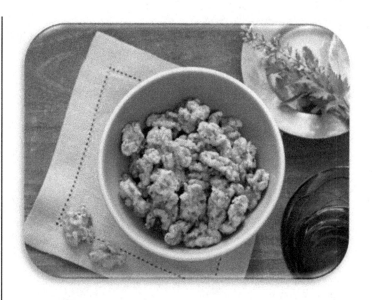

Instructions:

1. Preheat oven to 250°F.
2. Mix all ingredients except egg white and walnuts.
3. Whisk the egg and stir in halved walnuts.
4. Combine walnuts and the cheese mixture.
5. Bake for 30 min on greased baking sheet. Serve cold.

Figs with Blue Cheese

Prep time: 5 min

Cooking time: 0 min

Servings: 2

Nutrients per serving:

Carbohydrates – 24 g

Fat – 4 g

Fiber – 3 g

Protein – 8 g

Sugar – 20 g

Calories – 120

Ingredients:

- 3 fresh figs
- 2 tablespoons blue cheese
- 1 sprig fresh rosemary, chopped
- 1½ tsp honey

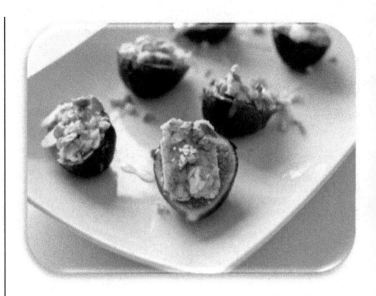

Instructions:

1. Halve figs.
2. Spread cheese on each half and top with fresh rosemary. Add honey to taste.

Festive Papas Tapas

Prep time: 10 min

Cooking time: 20 min

Servings: 6

Nutrients per serving:

Carbohydrates – 14 g

Fat – 5 g

Fiber – 1 g

Protein – 2 g

Sugar – 20 g

Calories – 100

Ingredients:

- 2–3 Yukon Gold potatoes, sliced
- 2 tsp extra virgin olive oil
- ¼ tsp pepper
- ½ tsp sea salt
- Bruschetta topping, to taste

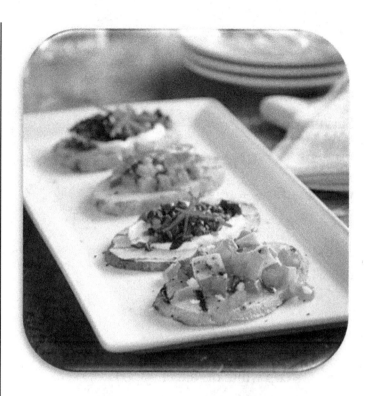

Instructions:

1. Preheat oven to 400°F.
2. Add a dash of salt and pepper, drizzle olive oil over each slice. Bake for 10 minutes on each side.
3. Top with your favorite topping, for example, Bruschetta topping.

Guacamole

Prep time: 5 min

Cooking time: 0 min

Servings: 10

Nutrients per serving:

Carbohydrates – 10 g

Fat – 13 g

Protein – 2 g

Calories – 160

Ingredients:

- 4 avocados
- ⅜ cup white onion, chopped
- ⅜ tsp salt
- 8 celery stalks, sliced into small sticks

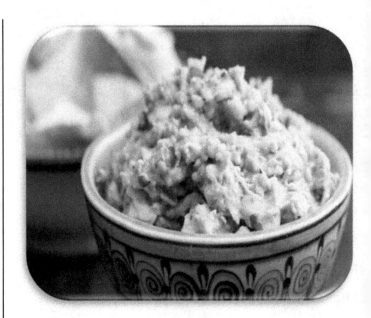

Instructions:

1. Mash 2 avocados into a smooth mixture.
2. Chop 2 avocados and stir into the smashed ones, adding onion and salt.
3. Serve with celery.

Evoo Cake

Prep time: 15 min

Cooking time: 40 min

Servings: 8

Nutrients per serving:

Carbohydrates – 45 g

Fat – 23 g

Fiber – 1 g

Protein – 5 g

Calories – 390

Ingredients:

- ¾ cup extra virgin olive oil
- 2 tsp baking powder
- 1½ cups flour
- 1 cup granulated sugar
- ¼ cup milk
- 3 eggs
- Salt to taste

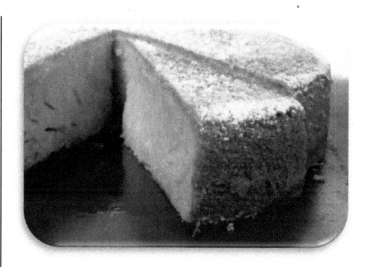

Instructions:

1. Preheat oven to 350°F and grease a cake pan.
2. Combine baking powder, flour, and ½ teaspoon salt.
3. Whisk together the eggs and sugar, then add in olive oil and milk gradually.
4. Combine wet and dry ingredients, pour into cake pan, and bake for 40 min.

PIZZA & PASTA

Mediterranean Pita Pizza

Prep time: 10 min

Cooking time: 20 min

Servings: 4

Nutrients per serving:

Carbohydrates – 40 g

Fat – 10 g

Fiber – 1 g

Protein – 16 g

Calories – 310

Ingredients:

- 4 whole grain pitas
- 1 cup tomato sauce
- 4 ounces mozzarella cheese, crumbled
- 4 cups vegetables, sliced
- 4 tsp extra-virgin olive oil

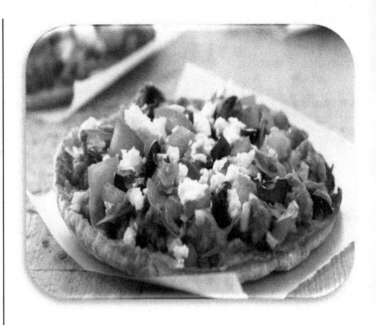

Instructions:

1. Preheat oven to 400°F. Put pitas on a baking sheet.
2. Spread tomato sauce over each pita and top with cheese and vegetables.
3. Bake for 15-20 minutes.

Pizza with Red Peppers & Anchovies

Prep time: 5 min

Cooking time: 15 min

Servings: 6

Nutrients per serving:

Carbohydrates – 11 g

Fat – 4 g

Fiber – 2 g

Protein – 4 g

Calories – 100

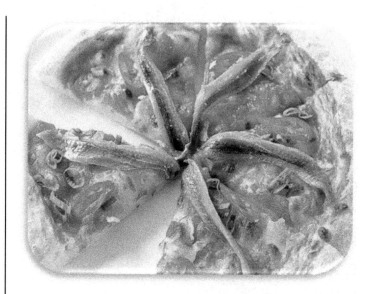

Ingredients:

- 6 anchovies
- 1 whole wheat pizza crust, pre-baked
- 1 Tbsp olive oil
- 13 ounces fire-roasted red peppers

Instructions:

1. Preheat oven to 350°F.
2. In a bowl, cover anchovies with milk and let rest for 5 minutes.
3. Sprinkle pizza crusts with olive oil. Cut the peppers and divide them between crusts. Top with the anchovies.
4. Bake for 15 minutes.

Rye Crispbread Pizza

Prep time: 10 min

Cooking time: 7 min

Servings: 2

Nutrients per serving:

Carbohydrates – 6 g

Fat – 4 g

Fiber – 5 g

Protein – 4 g

Calories – 110

Ingredients:

- 8 slices rye crispbread
- 8 cherry tomatoes
- 8 mini mozzarellas
- 4 ounces pizza cheese, grated
- 1 Tbsp olive oil
- 2 Tbsp basil, chopped

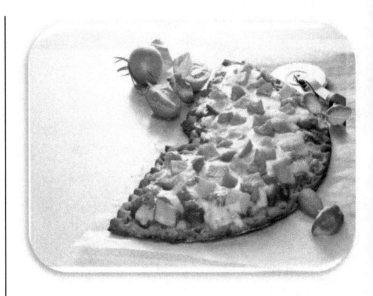

Instructions:

1. Preheat oven to 400°F.
2. Top crispbreads with olive oil, cheese, tomatoes, and basil.
3. Bake for 7 minutes or until the color has changed.

Feta & Beans Pizza

Prep time: 10 min

Cooking time: 20 min

Servings: 2

Nutrients per serving:

Carbohydrates – 49 g

Fat – 11 g

Fiber – 8 g

Protein – 15 g

Calories – 320

Ingredients:

- 1 Lavash
- 4 Tbsp Feta
- ½ cup fire-roasted red peppers, diced
- ½ cup black beans, cooked
- ½ cup cheddar cheese, grated

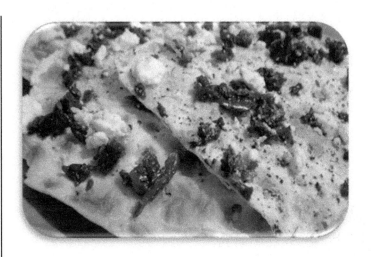

Instructions:

1. Preheat oven to 350°F.
2. Make 2 pizza crusts from Lavash. Put them in the oven for 5 minutes to brown. Let cool.
3. Top pizza crusts with remaining ingredients.
4. Bake for 10 minutes.

Pasta with Peas

Prep time: 10 min

Cooking time: 10 min

Servings: 4

Nutrients per serving:

Carbohydrates – 73 g

Fat – 11 g

Fiber – 10 g

Protein – 20 g

Calories – 480

Ingredients:

- 2 eggs
- 1 cup frozen peas
- ½ cup Parmigiano-Reggiano cheese, grated
- 12 ounces linguini
- 1 Tbsp olive oil
- 1 onion, sliced
- Salt & pepper, to taste

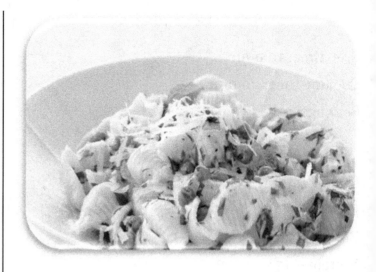

Instructions:

1. Prepare linguini according to package.
2. Whisk eggs and mix in cheese.
3. Sauté onion in olive oil, then stir in peas. Add pasta to pan.
4. Add egg mixture to the pasta and cook for another 2 min. Season with salt and pepper.
5. Serve hot.

Pasta with Roasted Vegetables

Prep time: 10 min

Cooking time: 20 min

Servings: 6

Nutrients per serving:

Carbohydrates – 11 g

Fat – 3 g

Fiber – 10 g

Protein – 2 g

Calories –95

Ingredients:

- 2 zucchini, chopped
- 2 cups cherry tomatoes, halved
- 14 ounce box farfalle
- ¼ cup parsley, chopped
- Olive oil

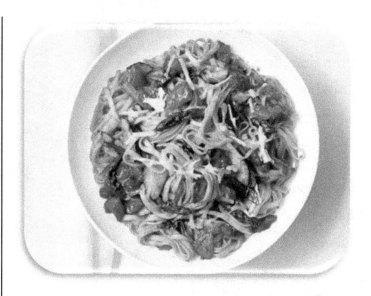

Instructions:

1. Preheat oven to 350°F.
2. Toss zucchini and tomatoes with olive oil and roast in oven for 20 minutes.
3. Cook farfalle according to package instructions. Combine with vegetables. Add parsley, and salt and pepper to taste.

Pasta with Prawns & Tomatoes

Prep time: 10 min

Cooking time: 20 min

Servings: 7

Nutrients per serving:

Carbohydrates – 51 g

Fat – 6 g

Fiber – 3 g

Protein – 15 g

Calories – 320

Ingredients:

- 1 pound pasta, preferably whole grain
- Black pepper, to taste
- ¾ pound cherry tomatoes
- ¾ pound raw prawns
- 1 Tbsp parsley, chopped

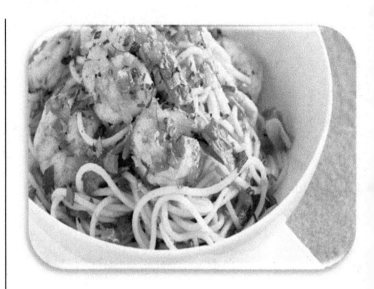

Instructions:

1. Cook pasta according to package. Then drain, but reserve a few tablespoons of the liquid.
2. Cook prawns and cherry tomatoes in a frying pan.
3. Add pasta to the prawns and stir.
4. Season with black pepper.

Sun-Dried Tomato Pasta

Prep time: 10 min

Cooking time: 20 min

Servings: 4

Nutrients per serving:

Carbohydrates – 80 g

Fat – 15 g

Fiber – 6 g

Protein – 20 g

Calories – 540

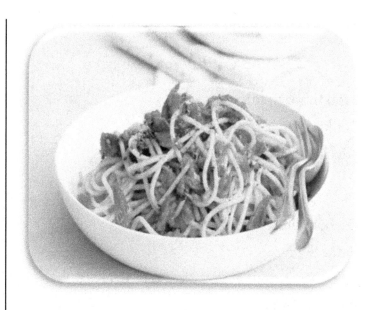

Ingredients:

- ¾ pound penne pasta
- 1 cup sun-dried tomatoes, sliced
- 1 cup red bell pepper, chopped
- 4 handfuls spinach leaves
- 2 cloves garlic, minced
- 2 Tbsp olive oil
- 1 cup Parmigiano-Reggiano cheese, grated
- Salt & pepper, to taste

Instructions:

1. Cook penne according to package instructions.
2. Combine all ingredients except cheese and add it to the prepared pasta.
3. Stir in cheese and mix well.

FISH & SEAFOOD

Baked Cod in Parchment

Prep time: 15 min

Cooking time: 30 min

Servings: 1

Nutrients per serving:

Carbohydrates – 35 g

Fat – 8 g

Fiber – 5 g

Protein – 25 g

Calories – 330

Ingredients:

- 1-2 potatoes, sliced
- 5 cherry tomatoes, halved
- 5 olives, pitted
- Juice of ½ lemon
- ½ Tbsp olive oil
- 4 ounces cod
- 20 inches long parchment
- Sea salt & black pepper, to taste

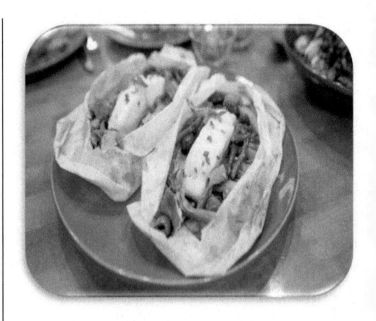

Instructions:

1. Preheat oven to 350°F.
2. Arrange potatoe slices on parchment paper.
3. Combine the tomatoes, olives, and lemon juice.
4. Put the fish fillet on potatoes and top with tomato mixture.
5. Fold the filled parchment squares into small packages. Bake for 20 minutes.

Provençal Salmon

Prep time: 10 min

Cooking time: 20 min

Servings: 4

Nutrients per serving:

Carbohydrates – 10 g

Fat – 30 g

Fiber – 3 g

Protein – 30 g

Calories – 420

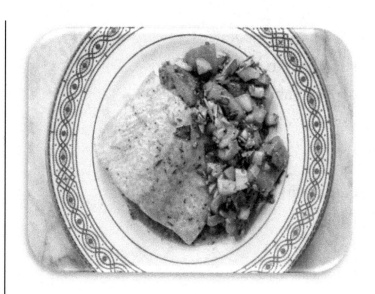

Ingredients:

- 8 ounces French mix of olives, peppers, and Lupini beans in white wine vinaigrette
- ½ pound Brussels sprouts, chopped
- 1 pound salmon
- 1½ Tbsp olive oil
- Parsley
- Salt & pepper, to taste

Instructions:

1. Preheat oven to 450°F.
2. Combine Brussels sprouts, olive mix, and olive oil.
3. Add salt and pepper to the salmon. Put all in a roasting dish.
4. Cook for 8-12 minutes.

Roasted Fish & New Potatoes

Prep time: 10 min

Cooking time: 35 min

Servings: 4

Nutrients per serving:

Carbohydrates – 315 g

Fat – 20 g

Protein – 41 g

Calories – 640

Ingredients:

- 3 Tbsp extra-virgin olive oil
- 3 Tbsp orange juice
- 3 Tbsp white vinegar
- ½ tsp orange peel, grated
- ¼ tsp dried dillweed
- 12 new potatoes, cubed
- 4 salmon fillets, skin removed

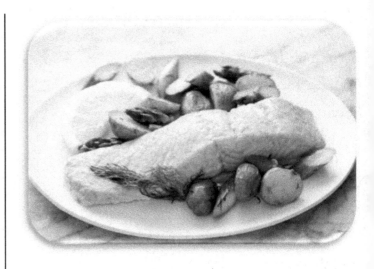

Instructions:

1. Preheat oven to 420°F.
2. Blend first six ingredients.
3. Sprinkle potato with 2 Tbsp of this mixture. Bake for 20 minutes.
4. Sprinkle fillets with remaining mixture and add to the potatoes.
5. Cook for about 15 min.

Pecan-Crusted Catfish

Prep time: 15 min

Cooking time: 10 min

Servings: 4

Nutrients per serving:

Carbohydrates – 15 g

Fat – 32 g

Protein – 32 g

Calories – 470

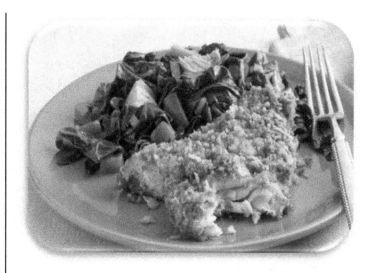

Ingredients:

- 1 egg
- 2 Tbsp water
- 4 catfish fillets
- ½ cup flour
- 1 cup pecans, chopped
- 2 Tbsp extra-virgin olive oil
- Salt & pepper, to taste

Instructions:

1. Combine egg and water. Put fish in mixture and let sit while preparing other ingredients.
2. Put flour on one sheet of wax paper, pecans on another.
3. Take each fish fillet from egg mixture. Coat one side of fish in flour, other in pecans.
4. Cook fillets in the skillet for 5 minutes on each side.

Spicy Salmon

Prep time: 20 min

Cooking time: 20 min

Servings: 4

Nutrients per serving:

Carbohydrates – 2 g

Fat – 10 g

Fiber – 1 g

Protein – 8 g

Calories – 270

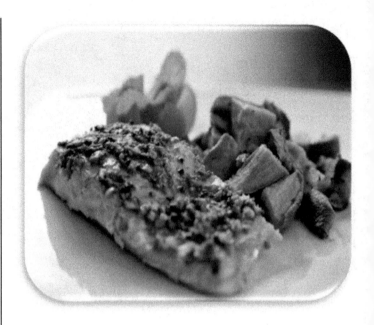

Ingredients:

- 4 cloves garlic, chopped
- 1 tsp red pepper flakes, crushed
- 2 Tbsp extra-virgin olive oil
- Juice of 1 lemon
- 4 salmon steaks
- ½ tsp sea salt

Instructions:

1. Mash garlic with salt, add other ingredients (except salmon) and make a smooth mixture.
2. Top fish with mixture and refrigerate for 2 hours.
3. Preheat the oven to 450°F. Bake for 20 minutes.

Shrimp Bucatini with Poblano & Zucchini

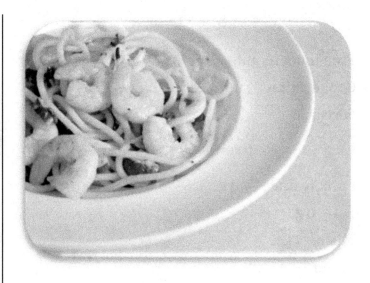

Prep time: 15 min

Cooking time: 35 min

Servings: 6

Nutrients per serving:

Carbohydrates – 60 g

Fat – 15 g

Fiber – 1 g

Protein – 23 g

Calories – 440

Ingredients:

- 1 pound bucatini
- ⅓ cup olive oil
- 2 poblano peppers, chopped
- 4 cloves garlic, sliced
- 2 zucchini squash, cubed
- 1 pound shrimp
- Juice of 1 lime

Instructions:

1. Cook the pasta according to package instructions.
2. In a skillet, cook poblano pepper and garlic with olive oil for 10 minutes. Stir in zucchini and cook for 15 minutes more.
3. Add the shrimp and cook for 3 minutes.
4. Season with salt, pepper, and lemon juice.

Skillet Shrimp

Prep time: 10 min

Cooking time: 9 min

Servings: 4

Nutrients per serving:

Carbohydrates – 5 g

Fat – 9 g

Fiber – 1 g

Protein – 24 g

Calories – 200

Ingredients:

- 1 pound medium shrimp, peeled & deveined
- 2 Tbsp extra-virgin olive oil
- 2 cloves garlic, chopped
- 1 tsp dried thyme
- 1 onion, sliced

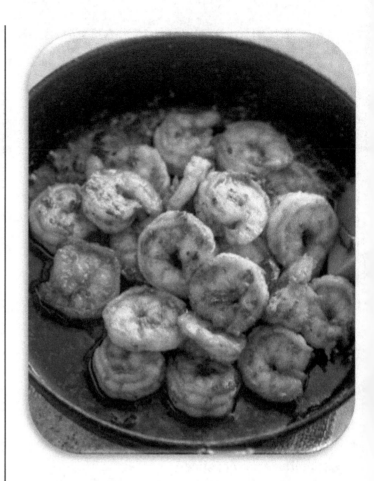

Instructions:

1. In a skillet, cook garlic, and onion in olive oil for 3 minutes.
2. Stir in the shrimp, thyme, salt, and pepper.
3. Cook for six min in the pan under the broiler (8 inches from the heat source).

Shrimp & Feta

Prep time: 10 min

Cooking time: 35 min

Servings: 4

Nutrients per serving:

Carbohydrates – 10 g

Fat – 20 g

Fiber – 3 g

Protein – 26 g

Calories – 320

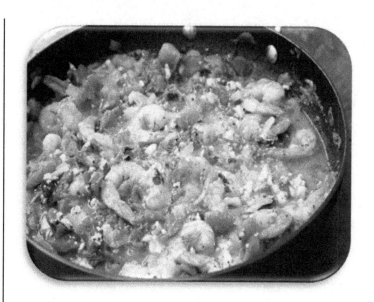

Ingredients:

- 1 onion, sliced
- 1 green pepper, sliced
- 2 cloves garlic, chopped
- 4 Tbsp olive oil
- 2 tomatoes, cubed
- 1 pound shrimp, peeled & deveined
- 8 ounces feta, cubed

Instructions:

1. Sauté the green pepper, garlic, and onion in olive oil for 5 minutes.
2. Stir in tomatoes and simmer for 15 min.
3. Add shrimp and feta. Season with salt and pepper to taste.
4. Cook for another 15 min.

MEAT & POULTRY

Spicy Chicken & Sesame Seed Balls

Prep time: 20 min

Cooking time: 10 min

Nutrients per serving:

Carbohydrates – 10 g

Fat – 210 g

Protein – 19 g

Calories – 290

Ingredients:

- 7-8 ounces chicken breast
- 1 clove garlic
- 1 egg white
- 1 ginger root, grated
- 1 tsp cornstarch
- 4 Tbsp sesame seeds
- 3 Tbsp extra-virgin olive oil

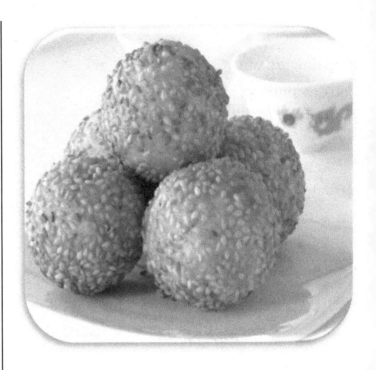

Instructions:

1. Blend first five ingredients in a food processor. Make balls out of this mixture.
2. Coat balls with sesame seeds.
3. Cook meatballs in olive oil in a skillet for 10 minutes.

Chicken & Wild Rice Quesadillas

Prep time: 1 min

Cooking time: 20 min

Servings: 6

Nutrients per serving:

Carbohydrates – 31 g

Fat – 22 g

Protein – 25 g

Calories – 430

Ingredients:

- 4 Tbsp olive oil
- 1 onion, chopped
- 1 garlic clove, minced
- 1 cup wild rice, cooked
- 2 cups chicken fillet, cooked, shredded
- 1 cup cheese, grated
- 6 tortillas
- Salt &0 pepper, to taste

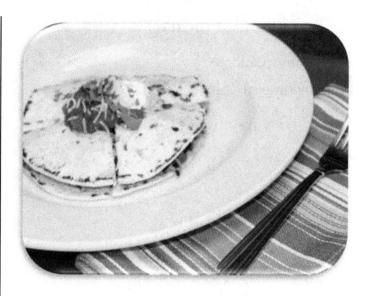

Instructions:

1. Cook garlic and onion in olive oil.
2. Combine it with the next three ingredients.
3. Divide this mixture between tortillas and top with cheese.
4. Fold tortillas in half and cook in a skillet until cheese is melted.

Quinoa Chicken Fingers

Prep time: 10 min

Cooking time: 10 min

Nutrients per serving:

Carbohydrates – 55 g

Fat – 44 g

Protein – 38 g

Calories – 770

Ingredients:

- 2 pounds chicken breasts, sliced
- 2 egg whites
- 1½ cups quinoa, cooked
- ½ cup breadcrumbs
- 2 Tbsp olive oil
- Salt, black pepper, paprika, to taste

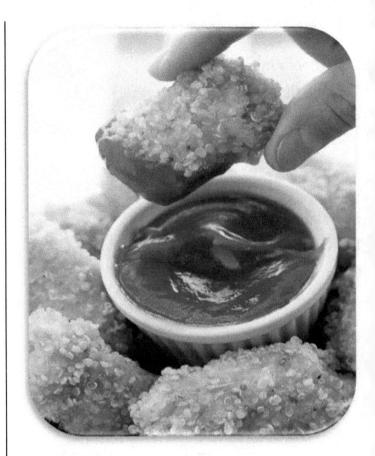

Instructions:

1. Season chicken with salt, pepper, and paprika.
2. Dip it into the egg, then coat with quinoa and breadcrumbs.
3. Cook the chicken in oil for 5 minutes on each side.

Grilled Lamb Gyro Burger

Prep time: 10 min

Cooking time: 10 min

Nutrients per serving:

Carbohydrates – 44 g

Fat – 28 g

Protein – 20 g

Calories – 470

Ingredients:

- 4 ounces lean ground lamb
- 4 naan flatbread or pita
- Olive oil
- 2 Tbsp tzatziki sauce
- 1 red onion, thinly sliced
- 1 tomato, sliced
- 1 bunch of lettuce, separated

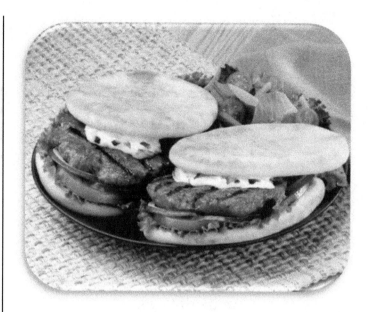

Instructions:

1. Grill meat for 10 minutes.
2. Toast naan bread, and drizzle with olive oil.
3. Top two of the halves of naan bread with meat and other ingredients. Cover with other halves and enjoy!

Chicken Stew with Peppers

Prep time: 10 min

Cooking time: 50 min

Servings: 8

Nutrients per serving:

Carbohydrates – 6 g

Fat – 22 g

Protein – 9 g

Calories – 291

Ingredients:

- 1 young chicken, divided into 8 parts
- ½ Tbsp extra-virgin olive oil
- 1 onion
- ½ cup dry wine
- 1 cup canned tomatoes
- 1 green pepper, sliced
- Salt & pepper, to taste

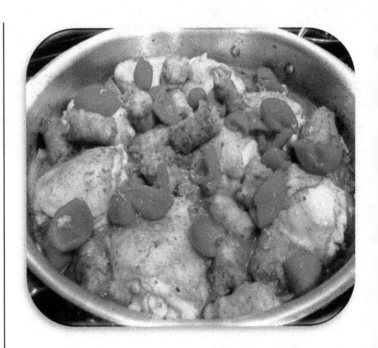

Instructions:

1. Sauté the onion in olive oil for 5 minutes.
2. Cook chicken with wine for several minutes. When the liquid is absorbed, add onions, tomatoes, and green pepper.
3. Season with salt and pepper. Cook for 30 minutes.

Italian Chicken with Noodles

Prep time: 15 min

Cooking time: 8 hours 20 min

Servings: 6

Nutrients per serving:

Carbohydrates – 33 g

Fat – 9 g

Protein – 29 g

Calories – 325

Ingredients:

- ½ pound chicken thighs
- 2 cups chicken broth
- 3 cups egg noodles
- 2 tsp thyme
- ½ tsp oregano
- 1 can tomatoes, chopped
- ½ cups carrots, sliced
- 1 onion, sliced

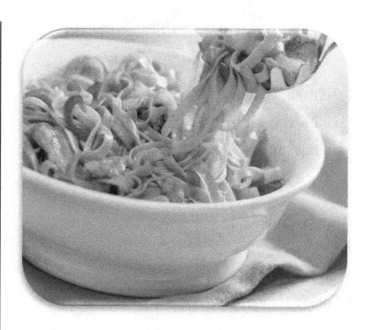

Instructions:

1. Put all ingredients except noodles in a pot and cook for 8 hours on low.
2. Add noodles, cook for another 20 min on high.

Mediterranean Slow Cooker Chicken & Potatoes

Prep time: 10 min

Cooking time: 4 hours 4 min

Servings: 6

Nutrients per serving:

Carbohydrates –43 g

Fat – 8 g

Protein – 45 g

Calories – 430

Ingredients:

- 4 chicken breasts
- 2 tsp Herbes de Provence
- ½ cup flour
- 1 tbsp extra-virgin olive oil
- ¼ pounds potatoes
- ¾ cup pearl onions, frozen
- 1 cup baby carrots
- ¾ cup chicken broth
- 8 ounces white mushrooms
- Salt & pepper, to taste

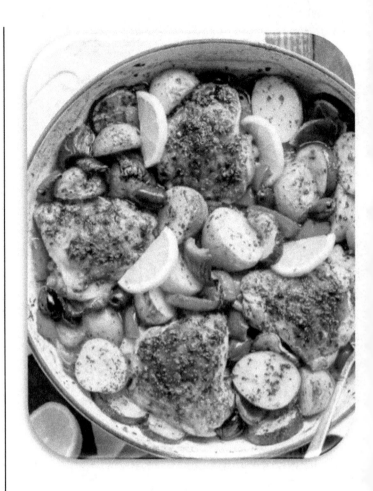

Instructions:

1. Dip the chicken breasts in herbs, then in flour.
2. Cook chicken 4 min in a skillet.
3. Put chicken and all other ingredients in a slow cooker and cook for 4 hours on high.

Chicken & Medjool Date Lettuce Wraps

Prep time: 10 min

Cooking time: 0 min

Servings: 4

Nutrients per serving:

Carbohydrates – 36 g

Fat – 12 g

Protein – 30 g

Calories – 370

Ingredients:

Dressing:

- ½ cup olive oil vinaigrette
- 4 Medjool Dates, chopped
- 2 cloves garlic

Salad:

- 2½ cups chicken, cooked, diced
- ⅔ cup Medjool Dates, chopped
- ⅔ cup red pepper, chopped
- ½ cup onions, sliced
- 12 lettuce leaves

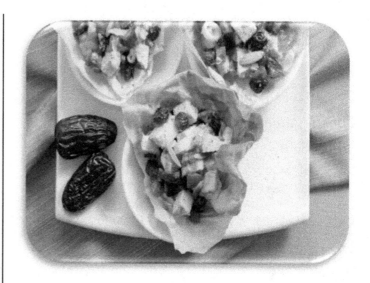

Instructions:

1. Blend all dressing ingredients and put in the fridge.
2. Combine first four salad ingredients and drizzle with dressing.
3. Divide the mixture between the lettuce leaves.

DESSERT

Chocolate Covered Figs

Prep time: 15 min

Cooking time: 15 min

Servings: 8

Nutrients per serving:

Carbohydrates – 55 g

Fat – 7 g

Protein – 4 g

Calories – 273

Ingredients:

- 1 ounce almonds
- 1¼ pound figs, dried
- 1 orange zest
- 1 tbsp ground cloves
- 4 ounces dark chocolate, melted
- 1 tbsp cinnamon

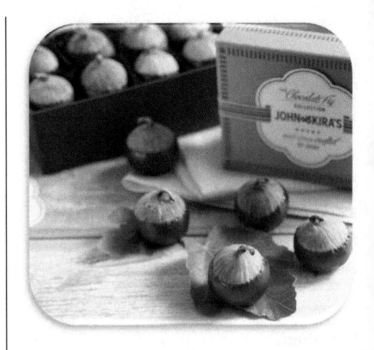

Instructions:

1. Preheat oven to 350°F.
2. Toast the almonds in the oven for 4 minutes.
3. Put an almond in the fig, and season with cloves and orange zest.
4. Bake figs for 10 minutes.
5. Stir cinnamon into melted chocolate. Dip figs into chocolate and let set.

Dried Figs with Ricotta & Walnuts

Prep time: 5 min

Cooking time: 2 min

Nutrients per serving:

Carbohydrates – 17 g

Fat – 8 g

Protein – 4 g

Calories – 142

Ingredients:

- 8 dried figs, halved
- ¼ cup ricotta cheese
- 16 walnut, halved
- 1 tbsp honey

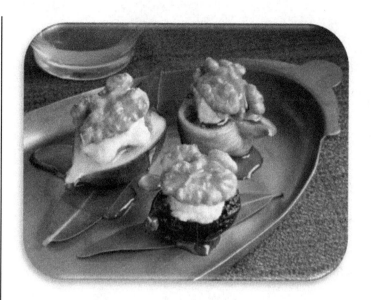

Instructions:

1. In a skillet, toast walnuts for 2 min.
2. Top figs with cheese and walnuts.
3. Drizzle with honey.

Summer Fruit Granita

Prep time: 20min

Cooking time: 40 min

Servings: 4

Nutrients per serving:

Carbohydrates – 40 g

Fat – 0 g

Protein – 14 g

Calories – 158

Ingredients:

- 1 pound ripe nectarines
- ½ cup sugar
- ½ cup water
- ¼ cup orange juice
- 2 tbsp lemon juice
- ½ cup raspberries

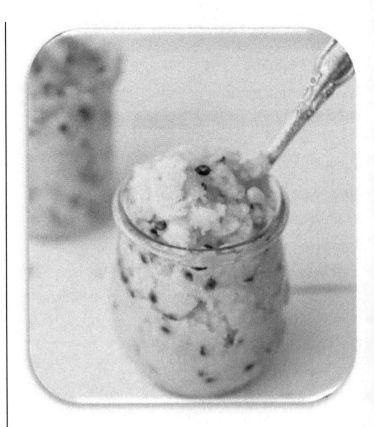

Instructions:

1. Boil fruit with sugar for 10 minutes.
2. Stir in raspberries.
3. Add juice and extra sugar, if needed.
4. Let this mixture freeze for 30 minutes. Using a fork, stir ice crystals, until it's granulated.

Banana-Strawberry Smoothie

Prep time: 5 min

Cooking time: 0 min

Servings: 2

Nutrients per serving:

Carbohydrates – 48 g

Fat – 8 g

Protein – 5 g

Calories – 330

Ingredients:

- 4 tbsp. rolled oats
- ¾ cup strawberries, sliced
- 1 banana
- 2 tbsp orange juice
- 1¼ cup fat-free yogurt
- 1¼ cup skim milk
- 1 tbsp flaxseed oil
- ¼ cup ice, cubed

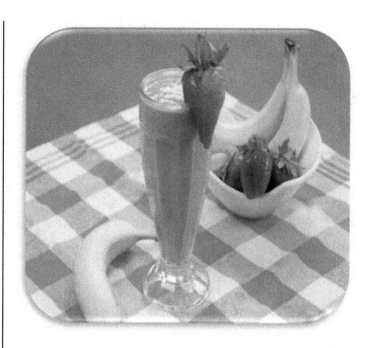

Instructions:

1. Blend all ingredients, making a smooth mixture.

Chocolate Mousse with Olive Oil

Prep time: 5 min(+ 20 min cool down)

Cooking time: 0 min

Servings: 6

Nutrients per serving:

Carbohydrates – 30 g

Fat – 38 g

Protein – 8 g

Calories – 490

Ingredients:

- 9½ ounces dark chocolate, melted
- ⅔ cup extra-virgin olive oil
- 3 Tbsp orange liqueur
- 7 eggs, separated
- ½ cup sugar, divided
- pinch salt
- orange zest

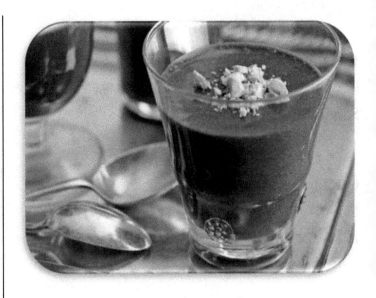

Instructions:

1. Mix the chocolate, olive oil, and liqueur in a bowl.
2. Wisk the egg yolk and half of the sugar. Combine it with chocolate mixture until smooth.
3. Stir in remaining sugar and salt.
4. Refrigerate for 20 min in small dishes before serving.

Date Porcupines

Prep time: 20 min

Cooking time: 15 min

Servings: 36

Nutrients per serving:

Carbohydrates – 8 g

Fat – 1 g

Protein – 1 g

Calories – 65

Ingredients:

- 1 tbsp extra-virgin olive oil
- 1 cup Medjool dates, chopped
- 1 cup walnuts, chopped
- 1 cup coconut, shredded
- 2 eggs
- ¾ cup flour
- 1 tsp vanilla
- ½ tsp salt

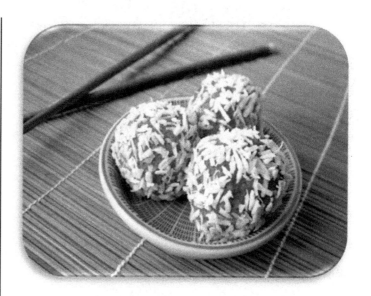

Instructions:

1. Preheat oven to 350°F.
2. Whisk the eggs with vanilla and olive oil.
3. Add in walnuts and dates, mixing well.
4. Mix in salt and flour.
5. Make balls out of this mixture. Coat them with coconut.
6. Bake for 15 minutes.

Medjool Date Truffles

Prep time: 20 min

Cooking time: 15 min

Servings: 10

Nutrients per serving:

Carbohydrates – 43 g

Fat – 12 g

Protein – 3 g

Calories – 265

Ingredients:

- 3 cups Medjool dates, chopped
- 12-ounce cup brewed coffee
- 1 cup pecans, chopped
- ½ cup coconut, shredded
- ¾ tsp orange zest
- 1 tsp. ground cinnamon
- ½ cup cocoa powder

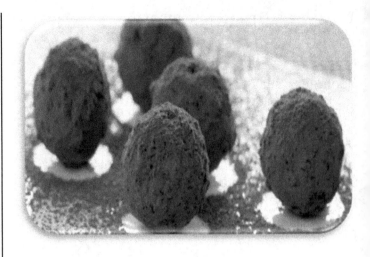

Instructions:

1. Soak dates in a warm coffee for 5 minutes.
2. Remove dates from coffee and mash them, making a smooth mixture.
3. Stir in remaining ingredients except for cocoa powder.
4. Form small balls out of the mixture. Coat them with cocoa powder.

CONCLUSION

Thank you for reading this book and having the patience to try the recipes.

I do hope that you have had as much enjoyment reading and experimenting with the meals as I have had writing the book.

If you would like to leave a comment, you can do so at the Order section->Digital orders, in your account.

Stay safe and healthy!

Recipe Index

Conversion Tables

VOLUME EQUIVALENTS (LIQUID)

US STANDARD	US STANDARD (OUNCES)	METRIC
2 tablespoons	1 fl. oz.	30 mL
¼ cup	2 fl. oz.	60 mL
½ cup	4 fl. oz.	120 mL
1 cup	8 fl. oz.	240mL
1½ cups	12 fl. oz.	355 mL
2 cups or 1 pint	16 fl. oz.	475 mL
4 cups or 1 quart	32 fl. oz.	1 L
1 gallon	128 fl. oz.	4 L

OVEN TEMPERATURES

FAHRENHEIT (°F)	CELSIUS (°C) APPROXIMATE
250 °F	120 °C
300 °F	150 °C
325 °F	165 °C
350 °F	180 °C
375 °F	190 °C
400 °F	200 °C
425 °F	220 °C
450 °F	230 °C

VOLUME EQUIVALENTS (LIQUID)

US STANDARD	METRIC (APPROXIMATE)
1/8 teaspoon	0.5 mL
¼ teaspoon	1 mL
½ teaspoon	2 mL
2/3 teaspoon	4 mL
1 teaspoon	5 mL
1 tablespoon	15 mL
¼ cup	59 mL
1/3 cup	79 mL
½ cup	118 mL
2/3 cup	156 mL
¾ cup	177 mL
1 cup	235 mL
2 cups or 1 pint	475 mL
3 cups	700 mL
4 cups or 1 quart	1 L
½ gallon	2 L
1 gallon	4 L

WEIGHT EQUIVALENTS

US STANDARD	METRIC (APPROXIMATE)
½ ounce	15 g
1 ounce	30 g
2 ounces	60 g
4 ounces	115 g
8 ounces	225 g
12 ounces	340 g
16 ounces or 1 pound	455 g

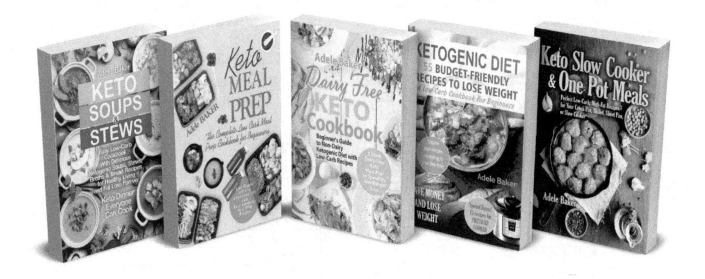

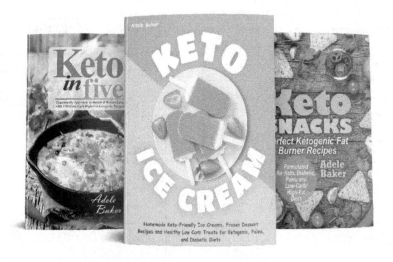

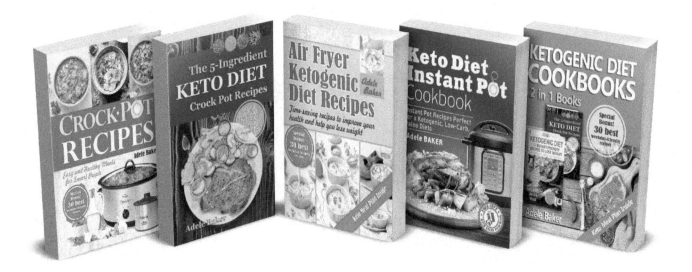

CPSIA information can be obtained
at www.ICGtesting.com
Printed in the USA
LVHW060034131120
671540LV00023B/308